COPD

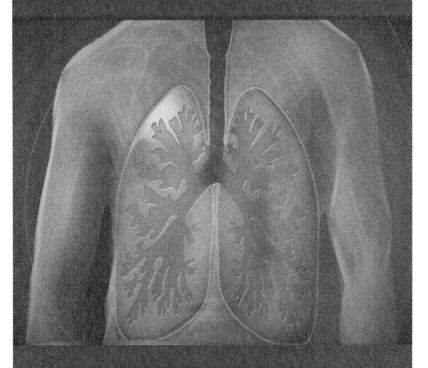

PETER YEXLEY

The boring legal stuff.

document, including, but not limited to, errors, omissions, or inaccuracies.

About the Author

Peter Yexley is qualified AET (formally Level 4 PTTLS) Education and Training, a knowledge-based teaching qualification and has tutored many accredited and regulated first aid and medical classroom courses including Emergency First Aid At Work (EFAW), First Aid at Work (FAW), Paediatric First Aid, First Person on Scene (FPoS), Administration of Penthrox, Canine First Aid, as well as a huge amount of bespoke courses including; Assisting The Paramedic, Catastrophic Bleed Management, Introduction to the range of tourniquets, Autoinjectors in Schools, First Aid in Schools, Emergency assessment and treatment at a search and rescue scene.

Plus, a growing list of online courses such as Understanding Medical Gases, Medication Administration, Enhanced Community First Responder, Emergency Trauma First Aid. First on Scene, First Responder at a Terror Attack.

As well as dedicating over a decade as a Community First Responder, responding to life-threatening 999 calls he also spent many years as a Team Leader Search Technician and Search & Rescue Medic for a Lowland Search and Rescue Unit, being called out only by police to assist them in the search for missing vulnerable persons.

As a keen and competitive, licenced, and certificated shooter, Peter not only entered competitions but provided event medical services.

He operates a small first aid service for events and is the founder of AoFAS – the Association of First Aid Services – www.AoFAS.org.uk

Peter is also author of over 20 eBooks, many are available on Amazon and Barnes & Noble. Mainly medical based information and lifestyle topics.

Contents

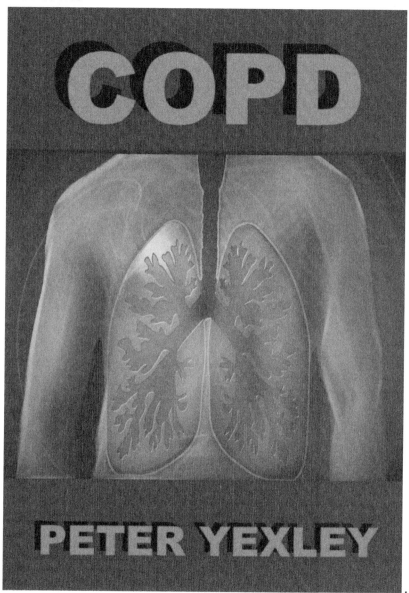

Introduction

Brief History of COPD

The history of CPOD goes back as far as the 1600s with Swiss-born physician, Theophile Bonet performing and recording over 3,000 autopsies on his patients. He first described the effects of emphysema on the lungs, noting that lungs were larger in patients who had suffered from emphysema.

In 1814, Charles Badham, a British Physician was the first person to use the term "bronchitis" to denote "inflammatory changes in the mucous membrane."

In 1821, Dr René Théophile Hyacinthe Laennec, a French physician and musician, and inventor of the stethoscope, known as the father of chest medicine, discovered the relationship between emphysema and chronic bronchitis.

He was the first to connect emphysema to aging and also the first to define emphysema as tissue damage in the peripheral air passages.

In 1837, Dr William Stokes of Dublin was the first person to use the term "chronic bronchitis."

in 1846, John Hutchinson, invented the spirometer, a tool still used today to diagnose and treat lung disease.

Moving into modern day, in 1959, there was a conference for medical professionals called the Ciba Guest Symposium and it was there and then that the full list of components for the definition and diagnosis of COPD was made.

Before it was officially called COPD, it was referred to as "chronic airflow obstruction" and "chronic obstructive lung disease."

However, it is believed that Dr William Briscoe is thought to be the first person to use the term COPD at the 9th Aspen Emphysema Conference in 1965.

In the 1960's, the term FEV1 was first used to measure expiratory flow.

According to Public Health England, around 25,000 people die each year from COPD in England.

Approximately 86% of those 25,000 deaths were caused by smoking.

The British Lung Foundation reported that up to 20% of people suffering with COPD have been affected by non-smoking-related causes.

BLF commented that COPD kills 30,000 people a year in the UK, just 5,000 less than the lung cancer. The UK's biggest cancer killer,

They also say "It is estimated that 2 million people in the UK have COPD but are currently undiagnosed. This means they can't get the support to give them the quality of life they deserve.

Up to 25% of long-term smokers will go on to develop COPD. – "

NHS Digital reported that COPD led to over 113,000 emergency hospital admissions in one year

GP figures revealed that more than 1 million people are living with COPD.

What is COPD?

Chronic obstructive pulmonary disease (COPD) is a lung disease.

Indicated due to obstruction of airflow through the lungs, interfering with normal breathing.

Before the term COPD was coined, we had more defined labels such as 'chronic bronchitis' and 'emphysema' but these are no longer used individually but included within the COPD diagnosis.

All too often people self-diagnose their lung condition as simply a "smoker's cough", whereas it is a life-threatening lung disease.

Even though COPD may be an umbrella term for Emphysema and chronic bronchitis, we need to take off the COPD 'shell' and look inside.

Emphysema is a lung condition that causes shortness of breath.

Patients who suffer from emphysema, the air sacs called 'alveoli' in their lungs are damaged. Let's focus on 'alveoli'.

Although the illustration below shows section C **alveoli with pneumonia**, the purpose of the whole image is for the reader to visualise a normal alveoli and indeed where they are found.

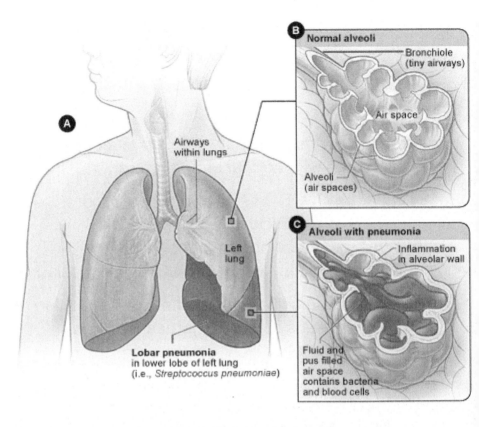

Alveoli play a crucial role in our respiratory system, their job is 'gas exchange', job description is to exchange oxygen and carbon dioxide molecules to and from the bloodstream.

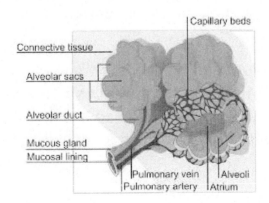

To gain a better understanding of where the alveoli live in our respiratory system, we could think of that system as a tree, branches, and twigs.

The 'respiratory tree' includes respiratory airways that lead into and out of our lungs as well as the lungs themselves.

The system creates a pathway of air starting from our nasal cavities (or oral cavity) down our pharynx, trachea, primary bronchi (right & left) into our secondary bronchi and tertiary bronchi then to bronchioles and finally the alveoli for gas exchange.

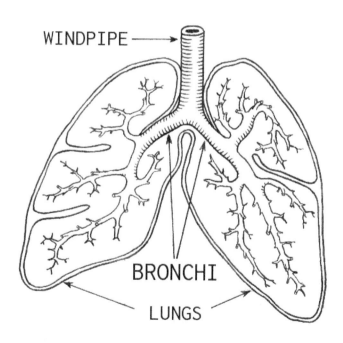

WINDPIPE ⟶

BRONCHI

LUNGS

Imagine tiny balloon-shaped air sacs or to fit in with the 'respiratory tree' visualisation, bunches of berries. They sit at the very end of the respiratory tree and like balloons or berries they are arranged in clusters throughout the lungs.

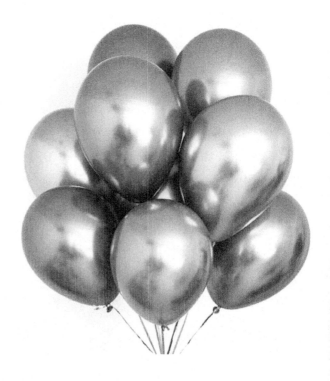

This part of the respiratory tree needs as much surface area as possible, so if it was say, one big balloon, it wouldn't have anywhere near the amount of surface area than lots of smaller balloons, and indeed if there were a lot more tinier balloons, there would be much more surface area.

As time passes in our life, those inner walls of the balloons (air sacs) weaken and rupture. This then creates larger air spaces instead of those many small ones, consequently reducing the surface area of our lungs. This in turn, reduces the amount of oxygen that reaches our bloodstream.

The damaged alveoli no longer work properly when we exhale, and old air becomes trapped. There is no room for fresh, oxygen-rich air to enter.

Many people who suffer from emphysema also have chronic bronchitis; this is inflammation of those tubes that transport air into our lungs (bronchial tubes) and leads to a persistent cough.

Emphysema and chronic bronchitis are two conditions that make up chronic obstructive pulmonary disease (COPD).

Both conditions narrow the airways making it very difficult to move air in and out as we breathe and rendering our lungs far less capable of taking in oxygen and expelling of carbon dioxide.

These airways have a lining of muscle and elastic tissue. A healthy lung has springy tissue between the airways like safety packaging and it grips and pulls on the airways enabling them to keep open.

With COPD, the airways are narrowed because of damage to our lung tissue therefore there is less pull on those airways.

In addition, mucus clogs up part of the airway or the lining becomes inflamed and swollen.

Smoking is the leading cause of COPD. There are treatments that may slow down the progression of COPD, but none as yet can reverse the damage.

More about COPD treatments later.

Is Asthma a COPD?

It is fair to say that both asthma and COPD have very distinct differences although they have similar symptoms, they can be identified as separate issues and the manner in which they present themselves is very different. Both are two of the most common kinds of lung disease.

Asthma Vs. COPD

Asthma is a lung disease that inflames and narrows the airways.

The vast majority of those who suffer from asthma are diagnosed at a very early age.

The disease itself is always present but not always displays the symptoms. What really happens is that the symptoms of asthma will come, and they will go.

This 'come and go' action all depends upon "triggers".

Well known triggers are:

- air quality
- dust
- dust mites
- environmental factors

- gastroesophageal reflux disease (GERD)
- inhaling cold, dry air
- mould
- pets
- physical activity
- pollen
- stress
- tobacco smoke
- upper respiratory infections

Research shows asthma to be genetic, however it must be said that a person might inherit the tendency to develop asthma, it does not necessarily mean they will suffer from it. In actual fact there is no clear reason why people actually develop it.

One of the biggest differences between COPD and asthma is that asthma is not altogether accepted as a progressive disorder. This means that a person's asthma could improve over a period of time and indeed some people can and do completely overcome it.

We mentioned earlier that COPD is an umbrella term used to cover chronic bronchitis, emphysema, or indeed a combination of both. Whilst COPD symptoms are remarkably similar to asthma symptoms, they are two totally different conditions and a few aspects that keep them from being under the COPD umbrella.

We know that people who are diagnosed with asthma are children, whereas most of those patients diagnosed with COPD are generally 40 years old or more.

COPD develops over time and lifestyle factors such as smoking are generally the cause.

COPD symptoms are milder than asthma symptoms, but the bigger difference is that COPD symptoms are constant.

COPD is progressive and become more serious over time. However, there are ways to keep it stable and manage the condition. More later on that.

COPD Symptoms

Because COPD is a progressive disease and is diagnosed later in life, symptoms all too often are not presented until significant lung damage has occurred, and even at that point, they are likely to worsen as time goes on. This is even more pertinent to those who continue to smoke or are exposed to smoke such as passive smokers or those that work in a smoky environment.

Signs and symptoms of COPD may include but not exclusively to:

- Breathlessness
- Chest infection
- Chest pain (advanced state, uncommon)
- Chest tightness

- Chronic cough that may produce mucus (sputum)
- Coughing up blood (advanced state, uncommon)
- Lack of energy
- Shortness of breath, especially during physical activities
- Swelling in ankles, feet or legs (advanced state)
- Tiredness (advanced state)
- Unintended weight loss (advance state)
- Wheezing

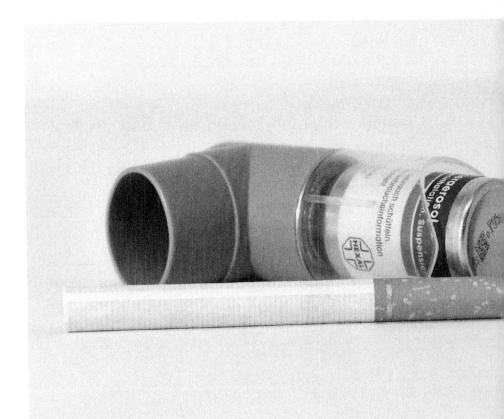

Be mindful that there are some conditions that may present similar symptoms, these include:

- Asthma
- Bronchiectasis
- Anaemia
- Heart failure.

NHS recommend that anyone experiencing persistent symptoms of COPD, particularly if you are over 35 and smoke or used to smoke, should contact their doctor.

COPD Testing

Diagnosis of COPD

If a person is showing signs and symptoms of COPD, their first point of call is to see their doctor. As well as enquiring about their symptoms, the doctor may ask them a set of standard questions before they are examined. The set of standard questions are likely to relate to the MRC Dyspnoea Scale. MRC is Medical Research Council and Dyspnoea means difficult or laboured breathing.

It is not compulsory for a doctor to ask, so the patient should not be concerned if they don't. However, in many cases it is clinically helpful to assess breathlessness using MRC grading of 1 to 5. This is a validated measure of disease severity irrespective of a patient's FEV1.

More on FEV1 later but in brief it is the quantity of air that a person can blow out in one second (that is what the 1 represents). If a person has healthy lungs and airways, they will normally blow out most of the air from their lungs in one second. FEV1 stands for **forced expiratory volume** in one second.

MRC dyspnoea scale

Grade	Degree of breathlessness related to activities

1	Not troubled by breathlessness except on strenuous exercise
2	Short of breath when walking in haste or up a slight hill
3	Walks slower than most people on the level, stops after a mile or so, or stops after 15 minutes walking at own pace
4	Stops for breath after walking about 100 metres or after a few minutes on level ground
5	Too breathless to leave the house, or breathless when undressing

Used with the permission of the Medical Research Council

Adapted from Fletcher CM, Elmes PC, Fairbairn MB et al. (1959) The significance of respiratory symptoms and the diagnosis of chronic bronchitis in a working population. *British Medical Journal* **2**: 257–266.

There is also a modified MRC Scale which is used in the GOLD guidelines and BODE - see Fletcher CM. Standardised questionnaire on respiratory symptoms: a statement prepared and approved by the MRC Committee on the Aetiology of Chronic Bronchitis (MRC breathlessness score). BMJ 1960; 2: 1662.

So, after asking how often the patient leaves their house and they declare that they are too breathless to leave their house, their grade would be 5 and it would be 5 too if they are breathless when undressing. More on this later.

Among the questions their doctor will ask if they smoke (or used to). Other questions relate to other factors that may increase their risk of COPD. These could include matter such as their exposure to dust or fumes at work, even a long time ago.

They may listen to your chest for sounds of wheezing or crackling when you breathe.

Depending on the results of the discussion and chest examination, the doctor may ask them to do a test called a **spirometry**.

What is spirometry?

Spirometry measures the quantity of air the patient is able breath out from their lungs and how fast they can blow it out.

The doctor will ask them to take a very deep breath and blow out as fast as they can into a mouthpiece,

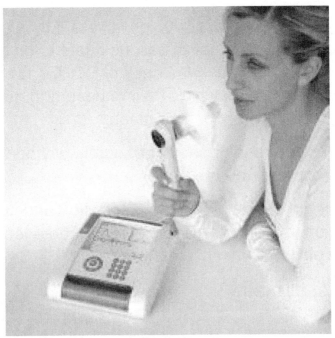

until no more air comes out.

A spirometry typical test takes around 10 to 20 minutes. If the doctor suggests bronchodilator responsiveness testing as well, then the whole test will take longer.

Bronchodilator responsiveness testing measures how well their lungs are working.

Before the test commences, the patient will be asked to take a medicine called a bronchodilator, this will help to widen their airways.

Then, using a breathing apparatus, the patient will be asked to take a maximum inhalation to fill their lungs to the most capacity possible, then release with maximum exhalation and continue to exhale for as long as possible to empty the lungs.

Following this first test the patient will be given the bronchodilator medicine. Finally, the spirometry test is repeated so as to determine how much the bronchodilator medication helped with breathing.

This is where the patient will be asked to take a deep breath and blow into the spirometer mouthpiece as hard as they can.

The measurement will tell their doctor if the symptoms could be due to COPD.

This may be the point where their doctor arranges a chest X-ray to see if the patient's lungs present any indications of COPD and at the same time to rule out any other lung diseases

A blood test may be required to check for anaemia or any signs of infection

Other tests for COPD

If the doctor diagnoses the patient with COPD, further tests may be required, such as:

- Blood test to check if the patient is deficient in alpha-1 antitrypsin. This is a deficiency that is an inherited disorder which may cause lung disease and liver disease.

- CT scan (computed tomography scan) to check the condition of the patient's lungs in greater detail. A CT scan is a medical imaging procedure that uses many X-ray measurements taken from different angles to produce "slices") of specific areas of a scanned object.
- ECG or echocardiogram to check the patient's heart

- Full lung function tests including peak flow measurement (how hard the patient can breathe out. This is to assess how well the patient's lungs are working

- Phlegm test. A test for infection on any phlegm the patient may be coughing up.

MRC Dyspnoea scale / MRC Breathlessness scale

Back in the 1940s the respiratory problems of Welsh coal miners were studied at the Medical Research Council Pneumoconiosis Unit and the researchers devised a serious of short simple questions. It allowed a numeric value to be embedded on each of the subject's exercise ability.

These questions were first published in 1952 and were soon after to become the MRC breathlessness scale. Now globally accepted as a clinical standard.

The MRC Breathlessness Scale

We looked at the MRC briefly, it comprises five statements but even though there are only five, they describe almost all of the entire range of respiratory disability.

Starting from no issues, which represents Grade 1, right up to complete incapacity, and that is Grade 5.

The questionnaire could easily be answered at home by the patient, prior to their visit to the doctor.

The questions are very straight forward and relate to everyday lifestyle activities, so, for instance, 'Are you short of breath when hurrying on the level or walking up a slight incline? If the answer is 'yes' then it represents Grade 2.

The MRC breathlessness scale is not intended to quantify breathlessness in itself but does quantify any disability associated with breathlessness and at the same time it identifies the point where breathlessness occurs when it should not, such as Grades 1 and 2, or indeed by quantifying the associated exercise limitation like those in Grades 3 to 5.

Grade	Degree of breathlessness related to activities
1	Not troubled by breathlessness except on strenuous exercise
2	Short of breath when hurrying on the level or walking up a slight hill
3	Walks slower than most people on the level, stops after a mile or so, or stops after 15 minutes walking at own pace
4	Stops for breath after walking about 100 yds or after a few minutes on level ground
5	Too breathless to leave the house, or breathless when undressing

Medication for COPD

Home Oxygen Therapy

The principle of oxygen therapy is that the patient breathes air that contains more oxygen than normal. This is delivered through a mask placed over the mouth and nose, or indeed a nasal tube (nasal cannula) positioned under the nose.

In some circumstances a tube is placed into the mouth and down the windpipe. Some patients may need a tracheostomy, where a tube inserted into an opening made in the front of their neck

The tube or mask is attached to a ventilator machine or oxygen cylinder.

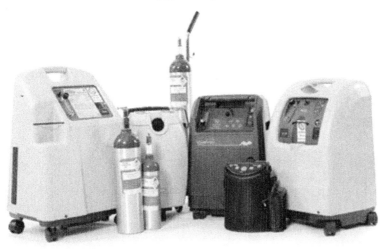

Picture courtesy of Bolton Pulmonary Fibrosis Support Group.

Some patients may only need oxygen therapy for short periods during the course of the day, it may be when they are walking around, even in the home. This is called ambulatory oxygen.

Others may need oxygen therapy for longer periods throughout the day as well as night.

Usually a doctor will refer the patient to a specialist clinic if feel that their symptoms can benefit home oxygen therapy.

It is not a 'cure' and should not be used to relieve breathlessness when a patient's oxygen levels are normal.

To assess the level of oxygen in a patient's blood, they may undergo a blood test and/or a pulse oximetry test using an oxygen sensor attached to their finger or earlobe.

Another method is the spirometry test where the patient is asked to breathe into a device that indicates how well their lungs are functioning.

Home Oxygen Devices
There are 3 types of home oxygen devices:

- Large oxygen cylinders
- Oxygen concentrator
- Portable cylinders

Large oxygen cylinders

These are likely to be prescribed when the patient only needs oxygen for a short time, for example, if they need to relieve sudden bouts of breathlessness.

Oxygen concentrator machine

An oxygen concentrator is a machine that concentrates the oxygen from a supply (usually ambient air), it removes nitrogen to supply an oxygen-enriched stream to the patient. These are recommended if the patient needs to have oxygen for most of the day, even when asleep.

They are about the size of an inkjet home printer and plugs into an electrical socket.

Portable oxygen cylinders

These are small, portable oxygen cylinders that are ideal for use outside the home. They are also called ambulatory oxygen.

Weighing about 2kg they are small enough to fit inside a small backpack or trolley and hold just under 2 hours' worth of oxygen.

They are not suitable for everyone.

There are approved suppliers in the UK that provide home oxygen services for the NHS. Each covers a certain geographical area so the patient will be advised as to their local approved supplier and they will also provide technical support.

Inhalers

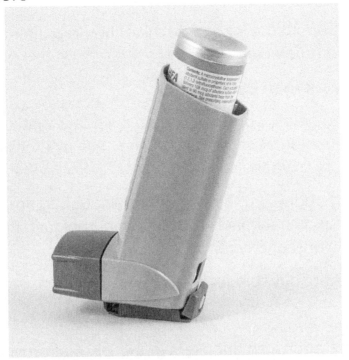

If COPD is affecting a patient's breathing, they are likely to be given an inhaler to deliver medicine directly into their lungs as they breathe in.

There are different types of inhaler for COPD patients:

Short-acting bronchodilator inhalers

Most patients who suffer with COPD, are likely to be prescribed a short-acting bronchodilator inhaler as the first treatment.

Bronchodilators were mentioned earlier, these are medicines that make breathing easier. They work by relaxing and widening the airways.

There are 2 types of short-acting bronchodilator inhaler:

1 Beta-2 agonist inhalers. (β_2) Examples are as salbutamol and terbutaline. Salbutamol, also known as Albuterol. It is marketed as the brand Ventolin as well as other brand names. Terbutaline is marketed under the brand name Bricanyl among other brands.

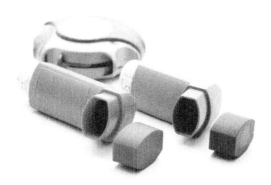

2. antimuscarinic inhalers – such as ipratropium, Ipratropium bromide is sold under the brand name Atrovent among others.

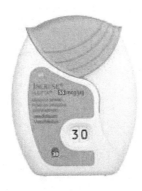

Short-acting inhalers are generally for use when a COPD patient is feeling breathless, and according to the directions prescribed

Long-acting bronchodilator inhalers

If a COPD patient experiences symptoms regularly throughout the day, their doctor may prescribe a long-acting bronchodilator inhaler.

They work just as short-acting bronchodilators do; however, each dose lasts for at least 12 hours, therefore they need to be less frequently but in accordance with the prescription.

There are 2 types of long-acting bronchodilator inhaler:

Beta-2 agonist inhalers. (β_2) The most common combination currently in use is fluticasone/salmeterol (brand names Seretide (UK) and Advair (U.S.))

Antimuscarinic inhalers – such as tiotropium (marketed as the brand name Spiriva), glycopyronium and aclidinium (marketed under the brand name Tudorza Pressair in the US, Eklira Genuair in the *UK*).

Newer inhalers contain a combination of a long-acting beta-2 agonist and antimuscarinic.

Steroid inhalers

Patients who still become breathless despite using a long-acting inhaler, or those who have frequent flare-ups may be prescribed a steroid inhaler as part of their treatment. These inhalers contain corticosteroids which can help to reduce inflammation of the airways.

Tablets

Doctors may prescribe tablets or capsules if a patient's symptoms are not controlled with inhalers.

Theophylline tablets

Theophylline is a type of bronchodilator (a medication that relaxes and opens the airways, or bronchi, in the lungs) that makes breathing easier, working alongside a preventer inhaler.

Doctors may recommend patients have regular blood tests whilst taking Theophylline tablets/capsules to check the level of medicine in their blood and help the doctor plan the appropriate dose to control symptoms and reduce the risk of side effects.

There are possible side effects that include:

- Nausea and/or vomiting
- Headaches
- Insomnia
- Heart palpitations that include noticeable pounding, fluttering or irregular heartbeats.

In some instances, a similar medicine called aminophylline is used to prevent and treat wheezing, shortness of breath, and difficulty breathing caused by asthma, chronic bronchitis, emphysema, and other lung diseases. The medicine relaxes and opens airways in the lungs, to make it easier to breathe.

Mucolytics

Mucolytics are used to treat phlegmy coughs. They reduce the thickness of mucous, and facilitate coughing it up, potentially increasing that coughing to expel the mucus.

Some examples of mucolytics include:

- Acetylcysteine (Fluimucil®)
- Bromhexine,
- Carbocisteine (Rhinathiol®)

Rhinathiol Promethazine® is a combination product of carbocisteine with promethazine.

If a patient has a persistent chesty cough with lots of thick phlegm, their doctor may prescribe mucolytic medicines to make the phlegm in their throat thinner and much easier to cough up.

Carbocisteine comes as tablets or capsules and is usually taken 3 or 4 times a day.

If carbocisteine does not help, or the patient cannot take it for medical reasons, there is another mucolytic medicine called acetylcysteine that is available in powder form and is mixed with water.

Be warned, Acetylcysteine powder has a rather unpleasant sulphur-like smell, very similar to rotten eggs.

Steroid tablets

A short course (probably 5 days) of these may be prescribed if the patient has a particularly bad flare-up to reduce the inflammation in your airways.

The 5-day course of treatment is generally recommended, because, long-term use of steroid tablets could cause side effects that may include:

- mood swings
- weakened bones (osteoporosis)
- weight gain

Where a longer course of steroid tablets is required, a COPD specialist must prescribe them.

Antibiotics

If a patient has signs of chest infection such as:

Breathlessness

Excessive coughing

Change in the colour of phlegm

Change in the consistency of phlegm

Their doctor may prescribe a short course of antibiotics

Pulmonary rehabilitation

Pulmonary rehabilitation, as the name implies is a is method of care that can help COPD patients improve abilities that they need for daily life. These abilities may have been lost because of disease, or even as a side effect from a medical treatment.

It is a specialised programme of exercise and education specifically designed to provide aid for patients with lung problems such as COPD.

Pulmonary rehab can help improve how much exercise a COPD patient is able to do before they feel out of breath, and it can help build self-confidence and emotional wellbeing.

Depending on your area and NHS availability, pulmonary rehabilitation programmes generally comprise 2 or more group sessions a week for at least 6 weeks. The programmes are provided by a variety of healthcare professionals, including physiotherapists, nurse specialists and dietitians.

A typical pulmonary rehabilitation programme includes:

- dietary advice
- education about COPD relating to the patient and their family
- bespoke physical exercise training to suit the patient's needs and ability, such as walking, cycling and strength exercises
- psychological and emotional support

Self-help for COPD

Much can be done in terms of self-help management of COPD.

It starts with COPD patients understanding their own condition including their own medications and how to manage any flare-ups which will make their everyday life much easier.

Light exercises

Probably the best and most natural way to improve the actions of a patient's lungs to their fullest potential is to keep active. It doesn't necessarily mean doing exercise but that can of course make a big difference.

There are some very sociable activities such as joining local social groups, perhaps walking, cycling even dancing. There is of course gardening and volunteering in the local community.

It may seem like a contradiction in terms but if a person with COPD is very breathless, exercising can be of great benefit to them.

Starting off lightly, if they are able to move around, may be a short walk for say 10 to 15 minutes, that's about one mile and back. If they did this, three to four times per week they will soon feel the benefit. Yes, they may soon get out of breath and that is OK, as long as they don't overexert themselves. It is all about taking things at their own pace and building up gradually when they feel ready.

If they are not able to move around, there are other ways to keep active such as stretching out their arms and twisting their upper body.

It is important not to allow physical limitations to be an excuse not to exercise and their doctor may be happy to refer them to a pulmonary rehabilitation programme.

A lot of people find exercise has helped them more than inhaled medication.

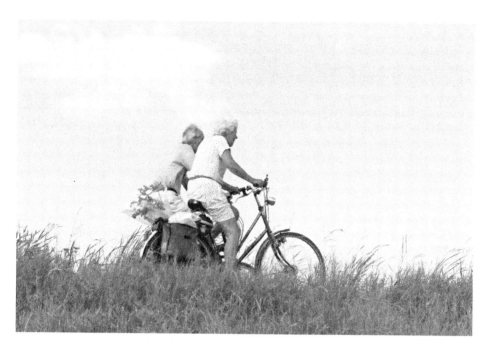

Giving up smoking

Many people believe that their COPD is just 'smokers cough' and far too many close their ears at the suggestions of stopping smoking, yet the most important thing that a smoker can do is to stop smoking.

It is likely that inhaling smoke is the cause of a person's COPD and indeed giving up smoking can relieve their symptoms as well as slowing down the progression of COPD, even if you've had it for a long time. A doctor will discuss ways in which they can help too.

Doctors have various options that may include nicotine replacement therapy or medicines to help people stop smoking, even contacts for support programmes.

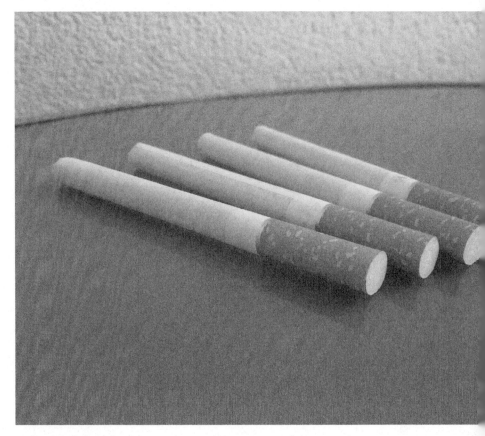

Eat healthy

Having a good eating plan isn't necessarily about losing weight, especially where COPD is concerned, it is about planning what to eat and balancing meals, these are crucial in health management.

There is no doubt that all healthcare professionals will advise their patients to make changes in their lives, this means eating healthy.

Let's not think for one moment that changing eating habits will cure COPD, it won't but it will go a long way feeling better.

COPD and good nutrition.

Let's look at why nutrition and managing COPD are linked.

Food is fuel, right? Breathing keeps us alive right?

Our body consumes food for energy as part of our metabolic process. During metabolism, food and oxygen are changed into energy and carbon dioxide.

All healthy diet plans bang the drum about carbohydrates, fat and protein, these are nutrients and our intake affect how much energy we have, also have how much carbon dioxide is produced.

We know that we exhale carbon dioxide as a waste product, but it is equally important to know that if there is too much carbon dioxide in our body, it can make us feel weak.

COPD patients need more energy because breathing requires more energy.

We use muscles to breathe and might need up to burn up 10 times more calories than those of a person without COPD, just to breathe.

So, there is the link between food and breathing.

Another top reason why we need good nutrition is because it helps our body fight infections. People that suffer with COPD often end up in hospital with chest infections, this is why it is important to reduce the risk of infection by following a healthy diet.

COPD or not, when someone is overweight, their heart and lungs have to work harder, this makes breathing much more difficult. On top of that the additional weight might well demand much more oxygen.

That would make us think that being underweight would be beneficial, however it would not, in fact it could make us feel weak and tired, as well as more likely to get an infection.

So if we accept that people with COPD use more energy to breathe than people without COPD and their breathing muscles might require up to 10 times the calories needed by a person without COPD, then we should accept the importance of consuming enough calories to produce sufficient energy in order to help prevent wasting or weakening of the diaphragm and other pulmonary (breathing) muscles.

If a COPD sufferer is underweight or overweight it is important that they ask their healthcare professional what a target, short term achievable goal should be.

Not their ideal weight but a target that they could achieve by taking positive steps.

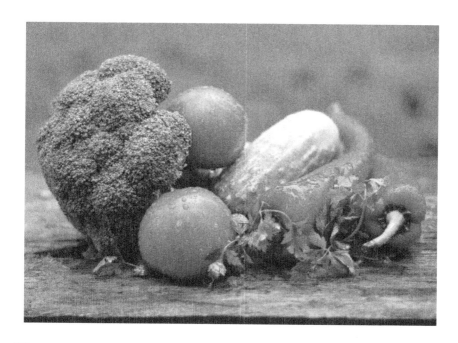

There is no need for fad diets, just good old fashioned, traditional food such as vegetables, fruits, peas and beans (legumes), whole-grain cereals, pasta, and rice. This comes under 'high fibre'.

Other element that sounds like a contradiction in terms is that fibre is the indigestible part of plant food.

So, if it is indigestible, how can it be good for us?

Fibre helps move food along our digestive tract, it can improve blood glucose levels, and might reduce the level of cholesterol in the blood.

To put it into perspective, to get enough fibre each day, all a person needs, to help get enough fibre would be a cup measure of All-Bran cereal for breakfast, a sandwich with two slices of whole-grain bread and 1 medium apple for lunch, For dinner 1 cup measure of peas, dried beans, or lentils.

Avoiding salt is a good thing because eating too much causes our body to retain too much water, and this in turn causes breathing to be more difficult. It is a good idea to use herbs instead of salt, even in cooking.

If a COPD patient is short of breath while eating or right after meals, try these simple tips:

Clear the airways at least an hour before eating.

Take small bites and chew food slowly, breathe deeply while chewing.
Put eating utensils down between bites.

Instead of three large meals, try eating five or six much smaller meals a day. It is a method that keeps the stomach from filling up excessively and the lungs have more room to expand.

Drinking liquids at the end of a meal is better because drinking before or during the meal might make a person feel full or even bloated.

Eat while sitting up to ease the pressure on your lungs.

Use pursed-lip breathing.

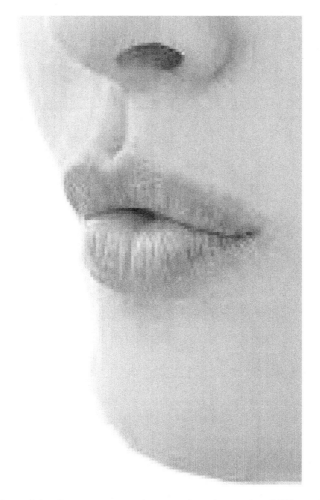

Food should play a very important part of life with COPD.

We have linked food with breathing, if we don't breathe, we die.

Eating a variety of foods from all the food groups will get the nutrients we all need.

Below is a list showing the recommended number of servings per day for a 2,000-calorie diet.

Grains

Whole-grain cereals, breads, crackers, rice, or pasta each day.

To get a measure of how much in a portion have 1 cup of cereal, or a half cup of cooked rice or pasta.

Eat 6 oz daily – one slice of bread is about 1 oz.

When it comes to breakfast cereals, below are the chosen top ones rated by the British Heart Foundation:

Porridge is a good healthy breakfast if it is made with low-fat milk or water and unsweetened.

Muesli that has no added sugar or salt and contains a good mixture of grains, fruit and nuts is a good choice but check the various brands for quality and contents, cheaper ones may not have as much fruit and nuts.

Shredded whole wheat cereal eaten with low-fat milk is the best choice of conventional breakfast cereals, it doesn't contain added sugar or salt, and it is high in fibre. A word of caution, the brands that contain fruit fillings, may contain added sugar, and the 'frosted' types will have added sugar.

Bran flakes are among the chosen few, along with malted wheat cereal and wheat biscuits such as Weetabix are high in fibre and may have sugar and salt added to them, so avoid adding sugar and consider adding fruits or berries for sweetness

Cornflakes or puffed rice served with low-fat milk, not the best choice but can be part of a healthy breakfast although they are low in fibre so not as good a choice as a wholegrain cereal.

Muesli WITH ADDED SUGAR is considered to be a healthy breakfast by many people but if you don't check that you are buying one with no added sugar or salt it can easily contain almost as much sugar as a bowl of frosted flakes. The upside is that we still get some health benefits from the nuts, grains and fruit but these are offset by the sugar, so be careful and choose no-added sugar muesli.

Sugar-frosted cornflakes (Frosties) are obviously high in sugar but also low in fibre as well and generally with added salt.

Granola of often thought to be a healthy breakfast but it isn't, because it is high in fat and sugar.

Vegetables

Which veg is best? Eat more dark green veg such as broccoli and also eat more orange veg such as carrots.

Add more dry beans and peas like pinto beans and lentils to your diet. They are cheap, very filling, and nutritious. As a guide two and a half cups of these per day is good.

Fruits

Eat a variety of fruit. Don't worry about getting fresh fruit in, frozen, canned or dried fruit is good too. Eat 2 cups daily

Be careful fruit juices. Whilst it is true that the proper pure 100% fruit juice is an excellent source of nutrients such as vitamin C and potassium, too much fruit juice can be an unwanted, unnecessary additional source of sugar and calories. Also be mindful that Juice doesn't contain the same fibre that raw fruits do.

Milk

Go for the green top low-fat or even fat-free milk, same with yogurt, and other milk products. Low fat or fat free is key.

For those who can't consume milk, lactose-free products or calcium-fortified foods or beverages are good options. 3 cups daily is ideal.

Meat

Take your time and read the packs of meat. Low-fat or lean meats and poultry is the best choice. When it comes to cooking, think before buy, can you; bake it boil it, or grill it? – no frying.

To vary protein in a diet, eat more fish, beans, peas. Nuts, and seeds are great for snacking too but everything in moderation.

Eat 5 and a half oz. daily.

Too tired to eat.

A lot of diets focus on weight loss, but many COPD patients feel too tired to eat properly and may resort to fast food or junk food.

Call on family and accept help from friends or neighbours to prepare foods. Don't be proud. Health is more important than pride. Check for eligibility to participate in the local Meals on Wheels service.

Select foods that are easy to prepare. Instead of buying whole cauliflower and broccoli, choose ready prepared frozen bags. If it takes a lot of energy to prepare food, cheat, save energy for eating, instead of being too tired to eat.

Prepare more than you need for one meal and freeze the rest, so you have a quick ready prepared meal for when you are too tired to eat another day.

Rest for a while before eating to enjoy and appreciate the meal.

It might be best suited to eat the main meal earlier in the day to store enough energy to last the day. Food is fuel for energy!

No appetite to eat

It isn't always a lack of energy, sometimes, poor appetite could be due to depression, and this can be treated. A visit to a doctor may well help and the appetite is likely to improve soon after treatment for depression.

Avoid non-nutritious beverages such as black coffee and tea. Black coffee contains no significant amounts of the macronutrients, fat, carbohydrate, and protein. Most traditional *teas* do not contain any significant amount of nutrients. Drinking too much tea and/or coffee could be filling and supress the appetite.

Going out for a walk or participating in light activity may stimulate the appetite.

It is all too easy to waste energy eating foods that provide little or no nutritional value.

We all like a bag of crisps or a chocolate bar but if they are not providing nutrition and spoiling an appetite, are they worth it?

Need to put on weight

A doctor or dietitian is a good starting point to discuss nutritional supplements that are more suited to the induvial rather than eating high calorie fatty food in an effort to put weight on.

The combination of exercise and supplements in the form of snacks, drinks or vitamins might be prescribed to eat between meals.

The right supplements will help increase calorie intake and achieve the right amount of nutrients that we need each day.

It is important that people who do take 'supplements' understand that they are to supplement meals and not replace them.

They are not a magic bullet for weight gain.

Aromatherapy and COPD

Extracts of plants have been used as medicines for thousands of years and many are still being rediscovered and often acknowledge by healthcare professionals and scientists as having healing properties than can work alongside prescribed medicines.

This extract from plants is called 'essential oil' and known for providing natural healing properties. Some can provide relief from COPD symptoms and indeed improve healthy breathing.

Before using any essential oils for COPD, consult a doctor to ensure there is no conflict with existing medicines.

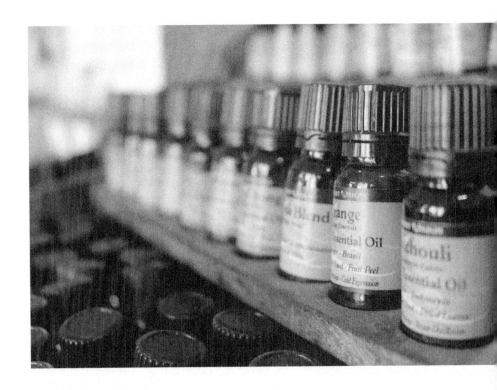

Eucalyptus

Eucalyptus has been used for centuries as natural therapy for better breathing and its oil could help with opening airways in COPD as well as treating inflammation.

COPD patients should be aware inhaling concentrated eucalyptus oil can cause lung irritation and make symptoms worse. It can also interact with medications.

It should be diluted with a carrier oil, these are vegetable oils, such as coconut oil, argan oil, jojoba oil or avocado oil. The ideal ratio is roughly five drops of eucalyptus per ounce of carrier. Some carrier oils are said to be odourless but will naturally have a faint smell of their product. Unlike essential oils, carrier oils don't evaporate

Look for a eucalyptus essential oil that is obtained through cold pressing because the oil is extracted by crushing the as opposed to heat extracted as this method may spoil the end-product.

Lavender

Lavender oil provides benefits to COPD patients because it acts as an antioxidant and boosts our immunity to fight against it. Lavender oil is known to have anti-inflammatory effects on the mucus lining of the respiratory system.

It is said that lavender oil can lower stress levels, this attribute is helpful as COPD can induce stress.

Myrrh

Myrrh essential oil boosts the immune system and reduces inflammation, used as far back as ancient times as a remedy for a host of ailments from minor pain to to leprosy. It is known to have antiseptic and anti-inflammatory properties.

Today myrrh oil is well in aromatherapy circles to relieve cold, cough, asthma, respiratory infections and ideal for treating COPD. Unlike eucalyptus, myrrh oil doesn't need to be diluted with a carrier oil unless the patient has sensitive skin.

Frankincense Essential Oil

Frankincense essential oil provides very similar benefits to myrrh. It has potent antimicrobial, antioxidant, and anti-inflammatory properties which help strengthen the immune system and fight COPD.

Peppermint

Peppermint essential oil offers a cool, minty, and refreshing aroma. That is used to alleviate asthma attacks and soothes breathing problems, so It can be of benefit to COPD patients because it acts as a natural decongestant.

Tea tree

Tea tree is considered beneficial for treating patients with COPD because it is known to relieve cold and cough symptoms. Follow proper aromatherapy instructions because tea tree oil is toxic if ingested.

Lemon

Lemon essential oil is a citrus oil that is known to keep infections at bay. Rich in vitamin C, and widely acclaimed to help fight against cough and colds.

Another benefit of lemon oil is it can soothe chest pains resulting from coughing.

Bergamot

Bergamot oil has antifungal and antibacterial properties that can help to fight against COPD. It also improves blood circulation, boosts immunity, and prevents infections, as well as alleviating pain and soreness caused by coughing during COPD flare-ups.

Bergamot belongs to the citrus family and is abundant in vitamin C.

Rosemary

Rosemary essential oil acts as a nasal decongestant and relieves breathing issues, thus, can be beneficial in treating COPD patients.

Chamomile essential oil is a sweet and fruity-smelling oil that has a calming effect on your senses. It promotes good sleep and patients can get enough rest to recharge their energy. The oil addresses other health benefits like skin rashes, arthritis, stomach aches, and digestive problems. Chamomile oil is used extensively in aromatherapy and manufacturing of other hygiene products. Never ingest chamomile oil.

Chamomile

Chamomile essential oil has a calming effect on our senses and promotes good quality sleep, so COPD patients may achieve sufficient rest to recharge their energy. Chamomile oil should not be ingested.

None of the above is meant to be directions or instructions on using essential oils for COPD but as a guide only.

How to Use Essential Oil For COPD

There are clearly many benefits in using some essential oils in aromatherapy for COPD patients, but it is important to know the right ways that these oils can be used to treat COPD patients.

There are a number of methods:

- **Diffuser method:**
  A diffuser is a device that is used to disperse essential oils into the atmosphere. Use a single or combination of oils to maximize the benefits of aromatherapy and may relieve COPD symptoms as well as lift the mood almost instantly.

  A tea candle is placed below a type of bowl that

would contain the essential oils and/or carrier oil,

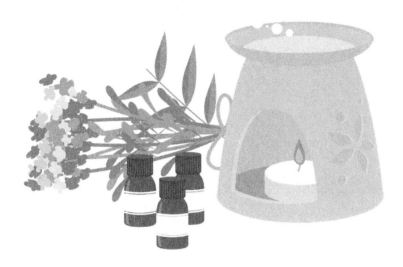

- **Chest rub:**
  As the name implies it is a form of vapour rub for the chest and different essential oils can be combined. A quantity of it can be made up and used for weeks to treat symptoms of COPD. Simply add a few drops of essential oil(s) to a specified measure of carrier oil such as coconut oil, argan oil, or jojoba oil. The ratio depends on the chosen essential oil and according to the instructions. This form of treatment will work as a decongestant, soothe muscle ache from coughing and relieve breathing difficulties.

- **Steam inhalation**
  Boil water, pour into a bowl or pan and add 1-2 drops of essential oil then inhale. An alternative method is to add the essential oils to a

humidifier. It is advised that the humidifier is cleaned well because the oils could cause build-up and impair the efficacy of the humidifier.

Vaccinations

These are not COPD vaccinations but the many recommended specific vaccinations, such as annual flu jabs and vaccinations against pneumonia that protect against serious and potentially fatal *pneumococcal* infections. COPD patients should ensure they are up to date to help to prevent flare-ups of COPD.

Managing COPD flare-ups

COPD, like many other diseases can be managed but not cured. With the right medication and self-help actions, it may be manageable, but from time to time there could be flare-ups in many different ways.

It is important that the COPD patient makes notes of these flare-ups; the date and time, describing the flare-up and the activity before it happened.

So, for example, the patient was taking out the wheelie bin at 8.30 then sat down, but within five minutes they felt breathless and dizzy.

This is the kind of information should be reported to the patient's doctor or healthcare team so that they can provide advice on how to recognise a flare-up and how to deal with it.

The incident may not be a flare-up but a consequence of an activity, so recognising it is important.

The patient may be given certain medicines for use when symptoms escalate. Advice on breathing techniques may also be given, these can help when the patient feels breathless.

Coping with breathlessness

Breathlessness can be very frightening as well as distressing, not just making it difficult to carry out our daily normal lives, but also affecting self-esteem as well as relationships.

It can add further feelings of anxiety, bringing on panics that may be difficult to control. Soon the patients get caught in a vicious circle making breathing worse.

COPD can affect basic daily activities, dressing and washing can be impossible, causing potential emotional distress, even anger, and that too can trigger increased breathlessness.

Reducing breathlessness

There are some activities that a COPD patient can do to prevent or reduce breathlessness.

Coping strategies, breathing and relaxation techniques are excellent activities to help reduce the distress of breathlessness and make breathing easier, but this doesn't that patients will not require further COPD treatments or medication.

COPD patients could rethink the way get dressed and undressed, some try and hold their breath in an effort to prevent them getting out of breath. This won't help even if they feel that it prevents breathlessness.

Sitting down when getting dressed, undressed, washing, and doing other tasks that can be done whilst sitting down such as preparing food.

It's a good idea to ask the doctor (hospital or GP) for a referral to an occupational therapist to gain advice about equipment and aids to avoid bending down and even standing up.

All the items that are used on a regular basis should be relocated so they are within easy reach as opposed to being too high up or very low down.

Good airflow is part of good breathing so opening windows and use of fans can help shift air around.

Wearing loose clothing, especially around the waist and chest can be beneficial.

Bathing and showers can be problematic for COPD patients and adjustments can be made, from using movable showerheads to redirect water from the face if it causes breathing difficulties. Using bathing chairs/stools. Don't have baths that are too hot. Wearing oxygen masks and breathing oxygen in the bath is OK and may help.

Use a towelling bathrobe after showering or bathing instead of a towel because less energy tis used than drying with a towel.

Pace activities throughout the day to conserve energy. Plan or set goals for activities and balance periods of rest with those of activities.

Sex and COPD

If COPD patients have an active sex life, they should try not to let it become a problem and try to manage around it.

Clearly a COPD patient needs to consider their breathing, equally their partner needs to take it into consideration.

Trying new activities or positions to enjoy sex despite COPD is good for a few reasons; the first being that COPD sufferers may find one or more perfect positions that enable them to enjoy sex and the other is it could be fun exploring those new positions and add another dimension to their sex life.

The obvious thing is to choose and use positions that are less likely to cause breathlessness or breathing difficulties over and above those that the COPD patient already suffers.

In this day and age, both partners in a relationship are expected to continue the relationship equally but with openness and willingness to learn and grow together as a couple. This means working and living around such conditions as COPD and not be isolated or deprived of pleasure in case it exasperates the problem.

COPD patients and their spouses could look at it as an opportunity to develop a new sexual relationship with their existing partner, explore new or even forgotten territory, learn new things and without being ashamed or embarrassed to suggest, as well as try them. It is important not use age as an excuse, if it is COPD that is the obstacle.

A good way to do this is to start dating again, not with other partners but with each other. Go on fun dates but tailored around COPD, cinema, events, gentle outings etc. Enjoy doing some things just as was done back in the day but be mindful of COPD.

Learning about each other's bodies again. Remember, time has passed, senses have altered, shapes have changed. So, start again by exploring each other, softly, slowly. Participants should let their partner know what is nice, what is good, really good and wow! This can be done by noise alone, no words necessary.

There are so many things a COPD patient and their spouse can do and try, it is important to experiment. Look at one of the various books about sexual techniques and positions, these will help you achieve a more thorough modern education on the art of sex with a few ideas that may be compatible with COPD.

Experiment with positions that may have no discomfort or distractions and worrying if a partner is having difficulties. It really does makes sense to try and test some positions until you find a few that will feel as comfortable as possible.

The following part is just an introduction or a reminder course to hopefully encourage you to pursue your lovemaking further.

WARNING SEXUAL CONTENT
DO NOT READ IF EASILY OFFENDED

Women on Top

There are quite a few positions for women to enjoy sex on top, some need good knees, other are fun simply instigating a session.

A lot men prefer to be on top of his female partner all

of the time and far too often the female never gets the opportunity to try different positions.

Many men like to be on top, it could be said for selfish reasons because it is simply more physically fulfilling him. However, there are those men who just are not secure enough in their own self esteem to let their partner to have what might be considered 'the dominant position'.

Many women prefer the sexual experience when they are on top as they can adjust speed and rhythm, so the lovemaking becomes much more rewarding for them. So, if the female suffers from COPD they can regulate movements to suit and if the male suffers and is below they are enjoying a less strenuous role. This applies to same-sex partners too.

It is of course a personal choice, and if a female has never had the opportunity to try it, the very least a caring, unselfish man can offer his partner is the opportunity to try and see how she likes being on top and even in charge of speed, depth and rhythm.

- **Cowgirl.** Think about a rodeo, pink cowboy hat not essential but could be fun! The man on his back with the woman facing him and mounted him.

  This position is good for both partners, because women get deep penetration and can control speed, rhythm, and her orgasm, it makes sensual contact with both the G-spot and the clitoris.

This also has the benefit of appreciating each other visually, eye contact can really improve climax, and cowgirl position creates a tighter sensation which is pleasurable for both.

- **Reverse Cowgirl**

  Women tend to enjoy reverse cowgirl, although some men with small penises may find it a little uncomfortable or unfulfilling, sometimes a tad awkward, or even impossible. However, it may be worth trying, the couple may find it satisfactory to each other,

  Once the woman is in position, she can lean forward, lean back, or sit upright, depending on personal preference and the management of COPD.

- **Chest on chest – tummy to tummy**
  This position simply involves the woman lying on her stomach on top of the man. Her legs are spread farther apart or held tight depending on personal choice. An excellent position if stamina is an issue, because it allows the woman to release pressure on the penis by spreading her legs, thus allowing for a longer encounter.

- **Chair position.**
  An iconic photo is that of Christine Keeler straddled naked across a cheap office chair by photographer Lewis Morley.

  The chair position is the male sitting down and the woman straddles his lap, facing him, It is important to note that the chair needs to be low enough to the floor so that the woman can touch the ground with her feet to steady herself as well as give her leverage.

  The best of two worlds is that this seated position is not only comfortable but great for stimulating those forgotten sweet spots

Man on Top

It is highly likely that you have already tried at least one of these positions and may be more simply because they are traditional positions where the man generally or traditionally takes the dominant sexual position.

Forget the top position being reserved for the man, it may have been in the past, but no longer. The choice of being on top is so the person in that position really takes control of the situation, perhaps for greater pleasure, perhaps to see their partner, there is clearly the point that a man or indeed a woman will simply prefer to have pleasure given to them. From a COPD perspective, there is that element of breathing control.

Spooning is best-known for its cuddle position and for many, it's more of a go-to position before and/or after sex.

For the best effect, the male cuddles up to the female's back. She nudges her buttocks back, pressing against him and he can penetrate her from behind or lift her leg so he can enter her from an angle. In simple terms it is doggie style, but with no pressure on knees, a great position for those suffering from COPD not to mention larger tummies.

Zen Pause.
With both partners lying on their backs, the female throws her nearest leg to the male over his body and finds an angle that allows entry. It is more of a side-by-side position and perfect for enjoying a close tender and relaxing moment with their partner. It is fun trying as well as aiding breathing control.

Not all sexual positions that may be compatible with COPD are described here and it really better for all parties to try various positions to see what works for them.

Finally, and above all, RELAX!

I hope you find the information in this eBook useful. In closing I have added some videos that are available in my YouTube channel. Please subscribe to the channel so that we can continue producing these free informational videos and if you would like to be notified of further free videos, click the Bell icon.

Kind regards

Peter Yexley

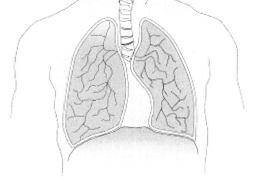

COPD
Pulmonary
Rehabilation

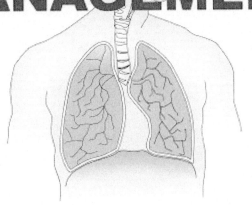

COPD
BREATHING MANAGEMENT

COPD
EXPLAINED

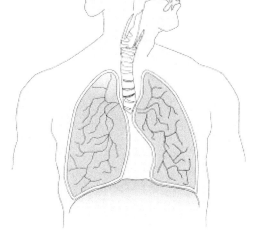

Printed in Great Britain
by Amazon